# NEVER GO HUNGRY

The Never Go Hungry Diet

Gary C. Fisher

Table of Contents

# CHAPTER 1

## YOUR BODY'S NATURAL CUES THAT IT NEEDS MORE FOOD IS HUNGER, WHICH IS WHY YOU'RE ALWAYS HUNGRY.

Your stomach may "growl" and feel empty when you are hungry, and you may also experience headache, irritability, or difficulty concentrating

However, not everyone is able to go several hours without eating before feeling hungry again.

This could be due to excessive stress or dehydration, a

diet deficient in protein, fat, or fiber, or a combination of the two.

*There are 14 causes of excessive hunger covered in this article.*

1. You are not getting enough protein Nadine United It is important to get enough protein to control your appetite.

Protein's ability to quell hunger may enable you to automatically consume fewer calories throughout the day. It works by decreasing the levels of hormones that cause hunger and increasing the production of hormones that indicate fullness.

If you don't get enough protein, you may experience frequent hunger pangs as a result of these effects.

One study found that 14 overweight men who got 25% of their calories from protein for 12 weeks had 50% less of a desire for late-night snacks than those who got less protein.

Moreover, those with higher protein consumption revealed more prominent completion over the course of the day and less fanatical contemplations about food.

Protein is abundant in a variety of foods, making it easy to consume enough of it. Every meal should contain a protein source to prevent overeating.

*Protein is abundant in animal products like meat, poultry, fish, and eggs.*

A few plant-based foods, such as legumes, nuts, seeds, and whole grains, as well as some dairy products like milk and yogurt, contain this nutrient.

Summary Protein regulates your hunger hormones, which helps you control your appetite. If you don't eat enough, you may experience frequent hunger pangs.

2. You are not getting enough sleep. Getting enough sleep is critical to your health.

Getting enough sleep is linked to a lower risk of several chronic illnesses, including heart disease and cancer, and it is necessary for the brain and immune system to function properly.

In addition, getting enough sleep is important for controlling appetite because it helps regulate ghrelin, the hormone that makes you want to eat more. Ghrelin levels rise when you don't get enough sleep, which can make you feel hungry.

In one study, 15 people who only slept for one night reported being significantly more hungry and choosing 14 percent larger portions than those who slept for eight hours.

Leptin, a hormone that makes you feel fuller, is also made by getting enough sleep.

It is generally recommended that you get at least 8 hours of uninterrupted sleep each night to control your appetite.

Summary: Lack of sleep has been linked to changes in hormones that control hunger and may make you feel hungry more often.

3. You are consuming an excessive amount of refined carbohydrates. Refined carbohydrates have been highly processed, and their fiber, vitamins, and minerals have been removed.

White flour, which is found in a lot of grain-based foods like bread and pasta, is one of the most common sources of refined carbohydrates. Refined carbohydrates also include baked goods, soda, candy, and foods made with processed sugars.

Your body quickly digests refined carbs because they lack fiber, which provides energy. Because refined carbs do not significantly increase feelings of fullness, you may experience frequent hunger pangs if you consume a lot of them.

In addition, consuming refined carbohydrates may cause rapid spikes in blood sugar. Insulin, a hormone that transports sugar into your cells, rises as a result.

When insulin is released quickly in response to high blood sugar, it quickly removes sugar from the body. This can cause hypoglycemia, a sudden drop in blood sugar.

If refined carbs are a regular part of your diet, you may experience frequent hunger pangs because low blood sugar levels tell your body that it needs more food.

Simply replace refined carbohydrates with nutrient-dense whole foods like vegetables, fruit, legumes, and whole grains to reduce your intake. These foods still have a lot of carbs, but they also have a lot of fiber, which helps control hunger.

Summary: Because refined carbohydrates lack fiber and cause fluctuations in blood sugar, eating too many of them can make you feel hungry.

4. Your diet is low in fat. Fat helps you feel fuller for longer.

This is in part because of its slow transit time through the digestive system, which means that it takes longer to digest and stays in your stomach for a long time. Additionally, consuming fat may cause the release of various hormones that promote fullness.

Therefore, you might feel successive yearning assuming your eating regimen is low in fat.

When compared to a group that followed a low carb diet, one study of 270 obese adults found that those who followed a low fat diet had significant increases in cravings for carbohydrates and preferences for high-sugar foods.

In addition, those in the low-fat group reported more hunger pangs than those in the low-carb group.

There are numerous supplements thick, high fat food sources that you can remember for your eating routine to expand your fat admission. Medium-chain triglycerides (MCTs) and omega-3 fatty acids, for example, have been the most extensively studied for their capacity to lessen hunger.

Coconut oil is the food that contains the most MCT, while fatty fish like salmon, tuna, and sardines contain omega-3 fatty acids. You can likewise get omega-3s from plant-based food sources, like pecans and flaxseeds.

Avocados, olive oil, eggs, full-fat yogurt, and other high-fat foods are additional sources of high-nutrient foods.

Summary if you don't eat enough fat, you may frequently feel hungry. This is because fat slows digestion and boosts hormone production that makes you feel fuller.

5. You are not properly hydrating yourself, which is critical to your overall health.

Drinking enough water has a number of health benefits, including improving exercise performance and promoting heart and brain health. Additionally, according to, drinking water helps maintain healthy skin and digestion.

When consumed prior to meals, water may also have the potential to curb appetite.

According to one study, 14 people who consumed 2 cups of water before a meal consumed almost 600 fewer calories than those who did not consume any water.

If you don't drink enough water, you might find that you often feel hungry because water helps you feel full.

It's easy to mistake feeling hungry for feeling thirsty. If you always feel hungry, you might be able to tell if you're just thirsty by drinking a glass or two of water.

Simply sip water whenever you feel thirsty to ensure that you are adequately hydrated. Consuming a lot of foods that are high in water, like fruits and vegetables, will also help you stay hydrated.

Summary if you don't drink enough water, you might always feel hungry. This is due to the fact that it suppresses appetite. Additionally, it's possible that you're mistaking hunger for thirst.

# CHAPTER 2

## INCREASE YOUR NUTRITIONAL ATTENTION

## 6. YOU MAY EXPERIENCE FREQUENT HUNGER PANGS IF YOUR DIET LACKS FIBER.

Eat a lot of foods high in fiber to control your appetite. Foods high in fiber take longer to digest and slow the rate at which your stomach empty's than foods low in fiber.

Short-chain fatty acids, which have been shown to promote fullness and the release of hormones that reduce appetite, are also influenced by a diet high in fiber.

It is essential to keep in mind that there are various kinds of fiber, and some are better at filling you up and preventing hunger than others. According to a number of studies, soluble fiber, also known as fiber that dissolves in water, is more filling than insoluble fiber.

Soluble fiber can be found in a wide variety of foods, including oatmeal, flaxseeds, and sweet potatoes, oranges, and Brussels sprouts.

A diet high in fiber is linked to a number of other health benefits, including a lower risk of heart disease, diabetes, and obesity, in addition to reducing hunger.

A diet high in whole, plant-based foods like fruits, vegetables, nuts, seeds, legumes, and whole grains will help you get enough fiber.

Summary: If you don't eat enough fiber in your diet, you might always feel hungry. This is because fiber helps you feel fuller and reduce your appetite.

7. You eat while distracted If you lead a busy life, it's possible that you frequently eat while distracted.

Distracted eating can have negative effects on your health, despite the fact that it may save you time. It is linked to having a bigger appetite, eating more calories, and gaining weight.

This is primarily because eating while distracted makes it harder to notice how much you're eating. According to, it prevents you from recognizing your body's signals of fullness as effectively.

According to a number of studies, people who eat while distracted are hungrier than those who eat without distractions at mealtimes.

88 women were instructed to eat while distracted or in silence in one study. When compared to those who ate without being distracted, those who were distracted felt less full and had a much stronger desire to eat more throughout the day.

Another study found that people who played a computer game to distract themselves at lunch felt less full than those who didn't. In addition, in a test that took place later that day, the distracted eaters consumed 48% more food.

You can try practicing mindfulness, limiting screen time, and turning off your electronic devices to avoid eating while distracted. You will be able to sit down and taste your food because of this, which will help you recognize your body's signals that it is full.

Summary: Because it's hard for you to tell when you're full, eating while distracted may be the cause of your constant hunger.

8. You do a lot of exercise

People who exercise often burn a lot of calories.

This is especially true if you train for marathons or engage in high-intensity exercise on a regular basis or for extended periods of time.

According to studies, people who exercise vigorously on a regular basis tend to have a faster metabolism, which means that they burn more calories at rest than people who exercise moderately or lead sedentary lives.

A 2014 systematic review of 103 studies, on the other hand,

found no consistent evidence to support an increase in energy intake while exercising. More randomized studies are required.

When compared to another day when they did not exercise, 10 men who participated in a vigorous 45-minute workout increased their overall metabolic rate by 37%.

According to another study, women who exercised at a high intensity every day for 16 days burned 15% more calories than those who exercised moderately and 33% more calories than those who did not exercise. For men, the outcomes were comparable.

There is some evidence that vigorous, long-term exercisers tend to have greater appetites than those who do not exercise, despite the fact that several studies have demonstrated that exercise is beneficial for suppressing appetite.

By eating more to fuel your workouts, you can prevent overeating while exercising. Increasing your intake of filling foods that are high in protein, fiber, and healthy fats is extremely beneficial.

Reduce the amount of time you spend exercising or the intensity of your workouts is another option.

It is essential to keep in mind that this mostly applies to avid athletes who frequently exercise at a high intensity or for extended periods of time. You probably won't need to consume more calories if you exercise moderately.

Summary: People who exercise frequently at a high intensity or for extended periods of time typically have faster metabolisms and larger appetites.

As a result, they might be hungry frequently.

9. You have consumed an excessive amount of alcohol. Alcohol is well-known for its ability to increase appetite.

Alcohol may inhibit hormones that reduce appetite, like leptin, according to studies, especially when consumed before or during meals. Thus, you might feel hungry frequently assuming that you drink a lot of liquor.

In one study, 12 men who consumed 1.5 ounces (40 milliliters) of alcohol before lunch consumed 300 more calories than those who consumed only 0.3 milliliters (10 milliliters).

Additionally, compared to those who drank less, those who consumed more alcohol consumed 10% more calories throughout the day. Additionally, they were more likely to consume foods high in fat and salt.

According to another study, 26 people who consumed 1 ounce (30 milliliters) of alcohol with a meal consumed 30% more calories than those who did not drink alcohol.

It's possible that drinking alcohol will not only make you

hungry, but it will also make it harder for you to exercise self-control and judgment. Even if you're not hungry, this could make you eat more.

It is best to consume alcohol moderately or completely to reduce its hunger-inducing effects.

Summary: If you drink too much alcohol, it can make you feel hungry more often because it makes fewer hormones that make you feel full.

10. You consume calories through liquids and solid foods in distinct ways.

If you eat a lot of soups, smoothies, meal replacement shakes, and other liquid foods, you might feel hungry more often than if you ate more solid foods.

The fact that liquids pass through your stomach more quickly than solid foods is one major reason for this.

Additionally, according to some studies (49, 51 Trusted Source), liquid foods do not have the same effect as solid foods on the suppression of hunger-promoting hormones.

Additionally, liquid meals typically require less time to

consume than solid meals. Because your brain hasn't had time to process signals that it's full, this may make you want to eat more.

In one study, people who ate a solid snack felt hungrier and felt less full than those who ate a liquid snack. Additionally, they consumed 400 more calories per day than the solid-food group.

Focusing on eating more solid, whole foods in your diet may help you avoid frequent hunger pangs.

Fluid food varieties don't affect keeping you full and fulfilled as strong food varieties do. Because of this, if you eat a lot of liquids, you might get hungry a lot.

11. You're stressed out too much Stress can make you eat more.

This is primarily because it raises cortisol levels, a hormone that has been shown to cause hunger and food cravings. As a result, if you have a lot of stress, you might always feel hungry.

In one study, 59 women who were under stress ate significantly more sweet foods and consumed more calories throughout the day.

350 young women's eating habits were compared in another study. Overeating was more common among those with higher stress levels than among those with lower stress levels. According to, girls with high stress levels also consumed more low-nutrient snacks like chips and cookies.

There are a lot of ways to lower your stress levels. Exercise and deep breathing are two options.

Extreme pressure is a justification for why you might be ravenous oftentimes, provided its capacity to increment cortisol levels in the body.

12. You are taking certain medications a side effect of some medications is an increased appetite.

Antipsychotics like clozapine and olanzapine, as well as antidepressants, mood stabilizers, corticosteroids, and drugs that stop seizures are the most common drugs that make people eat more.

Additionally, it is known that some diabetes medications, such as insulin, insulin secretagogues, and thiazolidinediones, can make you feel fuller.

Anecdotal evidence suggests that birth control pills can increase appetite, but solid scientific research does not back this up.

Talk to your doctor about other treatment options if you think that your frequent hunger is caused by medications. Alternative medications that don't make you hungry may exist.

Summary: As a side effect, some medications make people eat

more. As a result, you might become frequently hungry.

13. You consume food too quickly the rate at which you consume food may influence how hungry you are.

Fast eaters, according to a number of studies, are more likely to overeat at meals and have a bigger appetite. Additionally, they are more likely to be overweight or obese.

According to one study involving 30 women, fast-food eaters reported feeling significantly less full than slow-food eaters and consumed 10% more calories at a meal.

In another study, the effects of eating habits on diabetics were compared. When compared to those who ate quickly, those who ate slowly felt fuller and reported feeling less hungry 30 minutes later.

When you eat too quickly, you lose the ability to chew and lose awareness, both of which are essential for reducing hunger pangs.

Additionally, eating slowly and thoroughly gives your body and brain more time to release hunger-fighting hormones and send signals that you are full

*Mindful eating includes these strategies.*

Slowing down your eating may be beneficial if you frequently feel hungry. This can be done by:

Taking a few deep breaths before eating, putting your fork down between bites, and increasing the amount of time you spend chewing your food are all good practices. Summary Eating too quickly doesn't give your body enough time to feel full, which can lead to an overabundance of hunger.

14. You suffer from a medical condition Frequent hunger may be a sign of illness.

First, diabetes is frequently feeling hungry. It usually comes along with other symptoms like excessive thirst, weight loss, and fatigue, which are caused by very high blood sugar levels.

Hunger is another symptom of hyperthyroidism, which is characterized by an overactive thyroid. This is because it makes too many thyroid hormones, which are known to make people hungry.

Hypoglycemia, or low glucose levels, may likewise build your yearning levels. If you haven't eaten in a while, your blood sugar levels may drop, which may be made worse by a diet high in sugar and refined carbs.

However, medical conditions like type 2 diabetes, hyperthyroidism, and kidney failure are also linked to hypoglycemia.

In addition, depression, anxiety, and premenstrual syndrome are all common causes of excessive hunger.

It is essential to consult your doctor if you have any suspicions that you may be suffering from any of these conditions in order to receive an accurate diagnosis and inquire about your treatment options.

Summary: If you are frequently hungry, you should rule out a few specific medical conditions because excessive hunger is a symptom of them.

Ultimately, excessive hunger is an indication that your body requires more food.

Hunger hormone imbalances can occur for a variety

of reasons, including an inadequate diet and certain lifestyle practices.

If you don't eat enough protein, fiber, or fat, all of which help you feel fuller and less hungry, you might feel hungry a lot. Extreme hunger is also a sign of chronic stress and insufficient sleep.

In addition, frequent hunger is known to be caused by some diseases and medications.

If you frequently feel hungry, you should look at your diet and lifestyle to see if there are any changes you can make to make you feel fuller.

It's also possible that your hunger is a sign that you aren't eating enough, which can be fixed by eating more.

You can also practice mindful eating, which aims to reduce distractions, improve focus, and slow down your chewing to help you know when you're full, if you're eating too quickly or are distracted at mealtimes.

There is a lot of evidence that bulk, or fiber, makes you feel fuller. Therefore, eat more whole grains, beans, fruits, and vegetables with higher fiber content. Additionally, these foods typically contain a lot of water, which makes you feel fuller longer.

2. Soup can quell your appetite. If you start your meal with a hot or cold bowl of vegetable-based soup or broth, you'll probably consume fewer calories overall. Avoid creamy or high-fat soups; instead, choose low-cal, high-fiber options like minestrone or vegetable-bean soups.

3. Gratify your appetite with a substantial salad. One study

found that eating a large, low-calorie, 100-calorie salad before lunch reduced calorie intake by 12 percent. At the point when they had a more modest plate of mixed greens (1 1/2 cups and 50 calories), they ate 7% less calories by and large. You can make similar servings of mixed greens utilized in the review: Throw romaine lettuce, carrots, tomatoes, celery, and cucumbers together, and top with sans fat or low-fat dressing. However, avoid the fatty salad! Even a small amount of a high-calorie salad can encourage us to consume more calories than if we ate nothing at all.

4. Keep your course. A little variety in our meals is beneficial and even beneficial to our health. Having multiple courses, on the other hand, can lead you in the wrong direction. Unless it is a low-calorie salad or soup of the broth variety, adding an additional course to a meal typically results in an increase in the total number of calories consumed for that meal.

5. An orange or grapefruit daily aides fend hunger off. Oranges and grapefruit, two examples of low-calorie plant foods high in soluble fiber, have been shown to speed up the satiety

response and maintain stable blood sugar levels. Better control over one's appetite may result from this. Oranges and grapefruits have the highest fiber content of the 20 most popular fruits and vegetables!

6. Get milk (or other low-fat dairy food varieties). A great way to get more of two proteins known to suppress appetite—whey and casein—is to consume more low-fat dairy products. Additionally, drinking milk may have particular benefits. Whey, the liquid part of milk, was found to be more effective than casein at reducing appetite in a recent study.

7. Related Include some carbs with fat, but not too much! A hormone known as lepton is released by our fat cells when we consume fat. When we're talking about fat in moderation, this is a good thing. A very low-fat diet has been linked to a lack of lepton, which can lead to an overindulgent appetite, according to research. Obviously, that is not what we want to do. However, this does not necessitate a high-fat meal. Obesity is more common in people who consume a high-fat diet than in those who consume a low-fat diet, according to research.

8. Take in some soy. Along with carbohydrates, soy beans provide protein, fat, and fiber. That alone would suggest that soybeans are more likely than most plant foods to satisfy us and keep our appetites under control. In any case, a new report in rodents proposes that a specific part in soybeans has unmistakable craving smothering characteristics.

9. Go wild. Because they contain protein and fiber, nuts help you feel fuller longer. You can snack on a few of these mineral- and vitamin-packed snacks between meals. But only a small

amount: Despite the fact that nuts contain healthy monounsaturated fat, they are high in fat.

10. You're eating too fast, so slow down. Your brain needs at least 20 minutes to understand that you should stop eating and that your stomach is officially "comfortable." You are less likely to eat too much if you eat slowly because the brain has time to catch up with the stomach.

**THE END**

www.ingramcontent.com/pod-product-compliance
Lightning Source LLC
LaVergne TN
LVHW010122170826
845678LV00012B/2548

*9798369691250*